Introduction

The kidney has a number of functions which include the excretion of waste products and the regulation of the chemical composition and acid-base balance of the body tissues. Perhaps its most obvious and familiar function is the ability to maintain the water content of the body, and thus the osmotic environment of the tissues, at a constant level. For many years the kidney was regarded as nothing more than a complex filter in which the glomeruli produced a filtrate from the blood plasma. The filtrate was modified as it passed along the tubules by the variable reabsorption of water and other substances, and also by excretion into the tubular lumen. On this basis, it was easy to understand the everyday observation that if one drinks a large quantity of water, the kidneys produce a great deal of pale almost colorless urine. On a hot, thirsty day, however, the urine is darker in color and is passed only in small quantities. Certain experimental findings, which will be mentioned later, made the original concept of kidney function untenable. Only recently have alternative theories been put forward as a result of the evidence produced by modern techniques.

Osmolality

Before describing the process of the production of urine by the kidney, it will be helpful to introduce the concept of osmolality—a useful method of expressing the concentration of the osmotically-active constituents of urine or any other solution. The osmotic pressure of a solution depends on the total number of particles (undissociated molecules and ions) per unit volume or mass of fluid. It is therefore convenient to use units which depend on the number of such particles present. For a substance which does not dissociate in solution, one *osmole* is a measure of the number of particles in 1 gram-molecule. A solution of 1 osmol/kg (or 1 gram-molecule/kg) exerts an osmotic pressure of 22.4 atmospheres. If the molecules dissociate at all, the number of particles will increase and 1 gram-molecule/kg will then exert a correspondingly higher osmotic pressure. For example, a solution of 1 gram-molecule/kg of sodium chloride, which dissociates almost completely, has an osmolality of nearly 2 osmol/kg. For biological purposes, the osmole is too large a unit and the milliosmole (mosmol, one thousandth of an osmole) is usually used. The concentration of osmotically-active particles in a solution may then be expressed in mosmol/kg water. A physicist would find this explanation

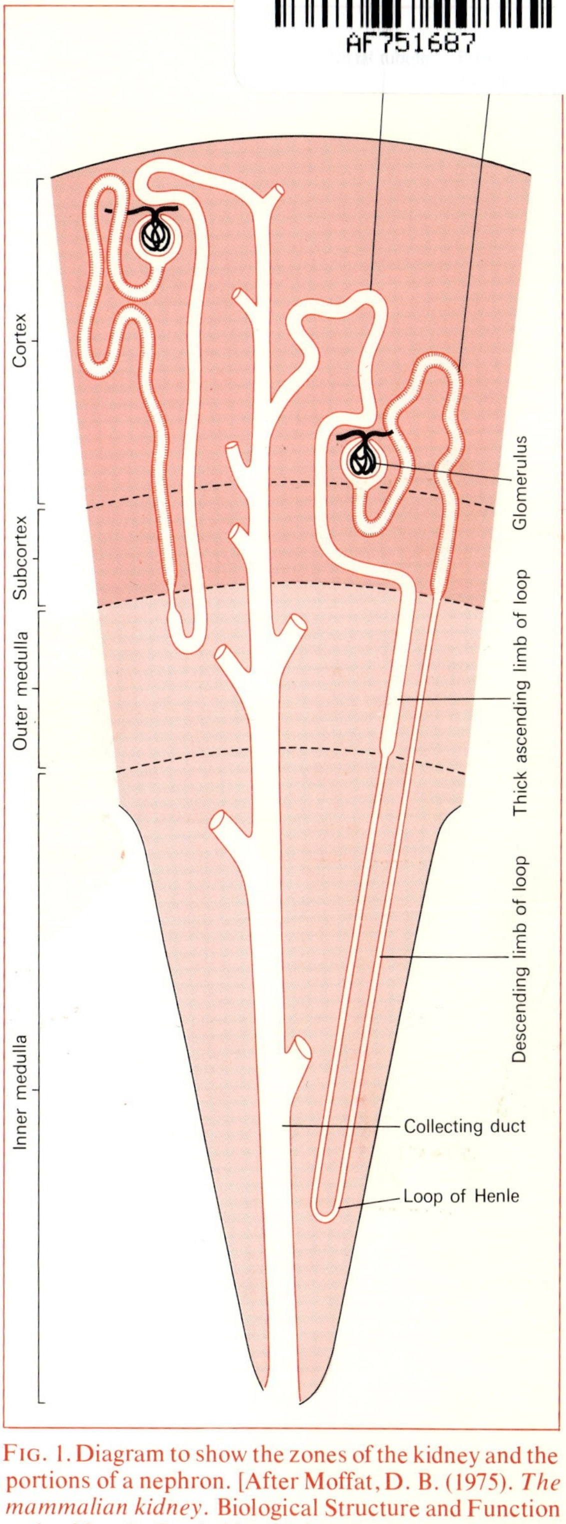

FIG. 1. Diagram to show the zones of the kidney and the portions of a nephron. [After Moffat, D. B. (1975). *The mammalian kidney*. Biological Structure and Function series No. 5. Cambridge University Press, London.] (By kind permission of Cambridge University Press.)

somewhat oversimplified, but it will suffice for present purposes.

Osmolality of urine

The osmolality of human blood plasma lies in the region of 300 mosmol/kg. Maximally concentrated urine may have an osmolality of 1400 mosmol/kg; it is 4 to 5 times as concentrated as plasma. In animals which live under arid conditions, even greater concentrations of urine can be obtained. The north African sand rat *(Psammomys)*, for instance, is able to attain the astonishing level of 6000 mosmol/kg. This tiny animal can therefore concentrate its glomerular filtrate, which has an osmolality in the region of 300 mosmol/kg (equivalent to an osmotic pressure of about 7 atmospheres), to a final urine with an osmolality equivalent to an osmotic pressure of almost 140 atmospheres.

Such an enormous change in concentration cannot be brought about by simple reabsorption of water from the lumen of the tubules. Thus, it became necessary to seek another explanation for the concentrating power of the kidney. Since about 1950, the importance of the renal medulla (Fig. 1) has been recognized in this respect. Prior to this time, the medulla was thought to be a rather uninteresting and inactive region compared to the cortex, and it was difficult to imagine any reason for the extraordinary course of the loops of Henle, which dip down for varying distances into the medulla before bending sharply back on themselves in a hairpin turn and returning to the cortex (Fig. 1). It is now known that the loops of Henle play an important part in producing a high osmolality in the tissues of the medulla which, in turn, is responsible for raising the osmolality of the final urine as it passes through the medulla in the collecting ducts.

The kidney is an organ in which structure and function are very closely correlated so that many deductions about its functions can be made from a detailed study of its structure. In the account which follows, the arrangement and structure of the various components of the kidney will be described; the significance of their structure in functional terms will also be discussed.

The nephron

The *nephron*, the basic unit of the kidney, consists of a *glomerulus* and a long *tubule* in which a number of sharply demarcated segments can be distinguished (Fig. 1). Each glomerulus consists of a cluster of capillaries that invaginate the hollow blind end

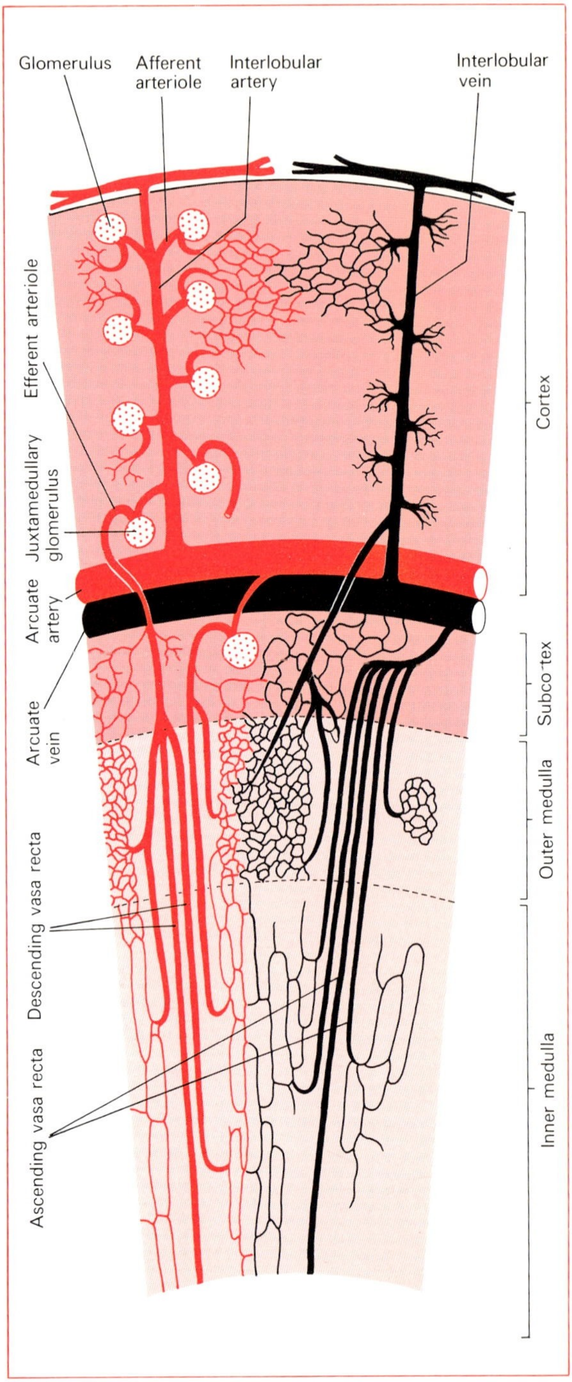

FIG. 2. Diagram to show the arrangement of arteries (left) and veins (right) in the kidney. In fact, the descending and ascending vasa recta are intermingled to form vascular bundles. [After Moffat, D. B. (1975). *The mammalian kidney*. Biological Structure and Function series No. 5. Cambridge University Press, London.] (By kind permission of Cambridge University Press.)

of a tubule, the thinned-out walls of which form the inner and outer layers of *Bowman's capsule* (Fig. 5). The cavity of Bowman's capsule leads directly into the *proximal convoluted tubule* which, after a tortuous course, has a short, straight segment in the subcortex. The tubule then becomes smaller and its wall becomes thinner as it passes down into the medulla for a varying distance to form the descending limb of the *loop of Henle*. Returning toward the cortex, the ascending limb abruptly becomes thick again, finally becoming the *distal tubule*. This comes into very close relationship with its own glomerulus and then, after a convoluted course, changes its structure gradually to become a *cortical collecting duct*. This changeover occurs earlier along the distal tubule than was previously thought, and the beginning of the cortical collecting duct is often mistakenly called the "late distal tubule." The cortical collecting duct joins with other similar ducts to form larger collecting ducts (common to many nephrons) which make their way through the outer and inner medulla, eventually opening onto the tip of the papilla along with numerous other major collecting ducts. In each human kidney there are about one million nephrons.

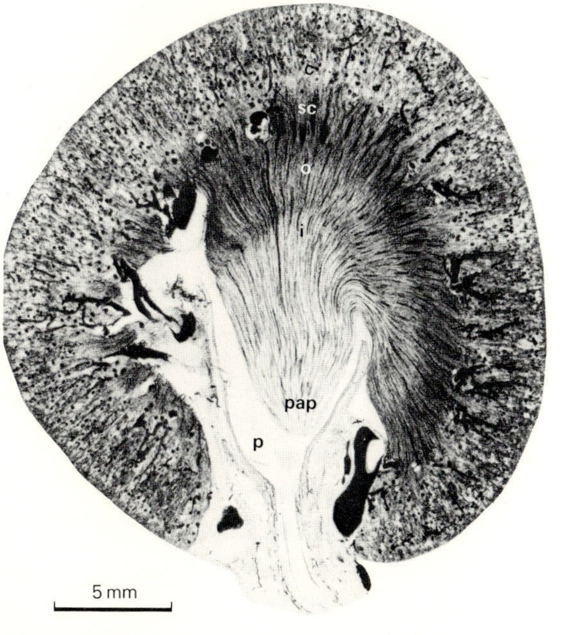

FIG. 3. Transverse section through a rabbit kidney, the blood vessels of which have been injected with India ink. Note the numerous glomeruli, which appear as small black dots in the cortex. Cortex (c); subcortex (sc); outer medulla (o); inner medulla (i); pelvis of kidney (p); papilla (pap).

The different portions of the nephron are so clearly demarcated that, in an appropriately prepared transverse section, the kidney can be seen to be divided into a number of zones, each of which contains particular segments of the nephron (Figs. 1 and 2). The outermost zone, the *cortex,* contains the glomeruli, most of the proximal tubules, the distal tubules, and the cortical collecting ducts. Inside the cortex lies the *subcortex,* characterized particularly by the straight part of the proximal tubules. The medulla is, itself, subdivided—the *outer medulla* containing the thin descending limbs of the loops of Henle, the thick ascending limbs and, of course, collecting ducts. The *inner medulla* contains the thin descending and thin ascending limbs of the loops of Henle and the large collecting ducts. Blood vessels, including a rich capillary plexus, are found in each zone. The most prominent vessels are the *arcuate arteries and veins* which lie between the cortex and subcortex (Fig. 2). The portion of the inner medulla which projects freely into the pelvis (or *calyx* in the case of the human kidney) is called the *papilla* (Figs. 3 and 4).

The structure of the human kidney (and of some of the larger mammals) is essentially similar to that of the rat or the rabbit, but it is a little more complex (Fig. 4). The cortex of the human kidney forms a complete surface layer but the medullary substance is subdivided into a series of units known as *renal pyramids*. The papillae of the pyramids project into subdivisions of the pelvis of the kidney which are known as *calyces* (sing.: calyx).

The glomerulus

The structure of the glomerulus is shown diagrammatically in Fig. 5. The *afferent arteriole,* which provides the blood supply to the glomerulus (Fig. 2) breaks up to form a network of anastomosing capillaries (Fig. 6) which reunite to form the outgoing or *efferent arteriole*. In the majority of the glomeruli this arteriole is very short and soon branches to form a network of *peritubular capillaries* around the cortical tubules, proximal and distal. The efferent arterioles of those glomeruli that lie nearest to the medulla (the *juxtamedullary glomeruli)* have a rather different distribution and this will be described later (p. 14). The glomerular capillaries themselves are closely surrounded by a layer of

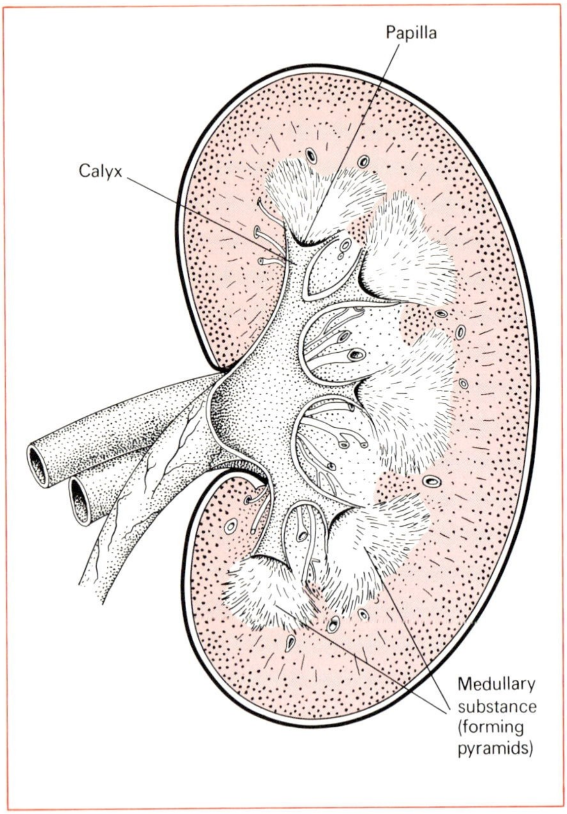

FIG. 4. Diagram of longitudinal section of human kidney to show how the medullary substance is subdivided into a number of pyramids.

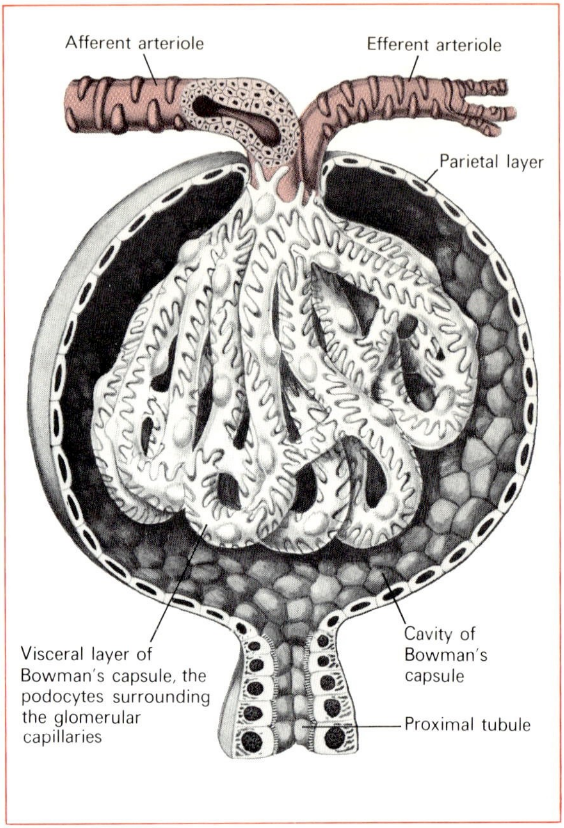

FIG. 5. Diagram of Bowman's capsule and the glomerular tuft of capillaries.

thin epithelial cells which form the inner, or visceral, layer of Bowman's capsule. At the vascular pole of the glomerulus these inner cells are continuous with the outer or parietal layer, which in turn is continuous with the much taller epithelial cells of the proximal tubule.

The function of the glomerulus is to produce a practically protein-free ultrafiltrate of the blood plasma. This enters the cavity of Bowman's capsule which is, of course, already full of ultrafiltrate, and passes into the proximal tubule. Although the glomerular capillaries are permeable to many proteins with relatively low molecular weights, they are almost completely impervious to the proteins which are normally present in blood plasma. The driving force behind the filtering process is the hydrostatic pressure of the blood in the glomerular capillaries. This has been measured in rats and is about 45 mm Hg. It is opposed by the pressure of the fluid in Bowman's capsule (about 9 mm Hg) and by the osmotic pressure of the proteins that are retained in the glomerular capillaries (about 25 mm Hg). The *effective filtration pressure* in the rat is thus only $45 - (9 + 25) = 11$ mm Hg (approx.). Small variations in the capillary or intracapsular pressures may therefore have a considerable effect on the glomerular filtration rate.

Nature of the filtration barrier

In many renal diseases, plasma proteins (especially albumin) may leak through into the glomerular filtrate. Thus, the structure of the barrier between blood and filtrate is of considerable importance and is worth examining in some detail.

It is first necessary to understand that, while the cells of the outer layer of Bowman's capsule form a complete layer of flattened epithelium (Fig. 5), those of the inner layer are of a much more complicated form, which is shown in Figs. 7 and 8. These cells, which are sometimes known as *podocytes* (literally "foot-cells"), are similar to starfish in shape, the "arms" or *trabeculae* each possessing a number of secondary or *foot processes (pedicels)*. The cells are arranged so that their trabeculae and foot processes embrace one or more capillaries; the picture is made more complicated by the interdigitation of the foot processes with those of the adjacent cells (Fig. 7). The tortuous cleft between the bases of the meshed foot processes is known as the *slit-pore* or *filtration slit,* since it is obvious that the glomerular filtrate has to percolate through this narrow cleft in order to reach the cavity of Bowman's capsule. In fact, the slit-pore is not an open space, for in a good electron micrograph one can see that it is closed by a very thin membrane (Fig. 9).

The capillaries themselves have a simple structure, consisting of an endothelium resting on a basement membrane. Except in the region of the nucleus, the endothelial cells are extremely thin and are perforated by large numbers of roughly circular openings or *fenestrations* which have a diameter of between 50 and 100 nm (Figs. 8, 9, and 10). Opinions differ as to the nature of the fenestrations. Some investigators have reported that they are not true pores since they are closed by a very thin membrane. This is certainly the case in the fenestrated vessels of other regions of the kidney (Fig. 19), but the majority opinion favors the view that no membrane is present in the glomerular capillaries. The apparent discrepancy in findings may, perhaps, be due to species differences.

In passing from the capillary lumen to the cavity of Bowman's capsule, the glomerular filtrate must traverse: (a) the endothelium, (b) the basement membrane, and (c) the slit-pores between the foot processes (Fig. 9). Somewhere within this composite membrane lies the physiological filtration system. This system allows water and small molecules to pass through, but retains larger molecules such as proteins. In spite of the importance of this membrane and much intensive research, the exact mechanism of filtration remains uncertain. A number of attempts have been made to investigate the problem by injecting substances of different molecular weights (which are electron-opaque or which can be rendered so by treatment with suitable reagents) into the bloodstream of animals. The endothelium seems to present no hindrance to the passage of protein molecules, which pass freely through the fenestrations. The principal barrier seems to be the basement membrane, which holds back molecules in the same size range as that of the plasma proteins. It is also possible that a further hindrance to the passage of large molecules may be provided by the membrane that closes the slit-pore, as well as, by the anionic *cell coat* that covers the foot processes.

The glomerular filtrate

The volume of filtrate produced by the glomeruli can be estimated by various indirect methods. The kidneys, between them, receive about one quarter of the total output of the heart, amounting to some 1300 cm^3 of blood per minute in man. This blood contains about 700 cm^3 of plasma (the rest of the volume is made up of cells) and of this, about 125 cm^3 per minute is filtered off by the glomeruli. This amounts to a total daily filtrate of something like 180 liters. Under normal conditions, the volume of urine produced is only in the region of 1.5 liters, so that about 178.5 liters of filtrate is (fortunately) reabsorbed by the tubules of the kidney. Experimental methods have shown that the greater part of the 125 cm^3 of filtrate produced each minute is reabsorbed by the proximal tubule, leaving only 15 to 20 cm^3/min to pass into the loops of Henle. This proximal tubule reabsorption is relatively constant and is therefore sometimes known as the "*obligatory reabsorption.*" The remaining 20 cm^3/min is reab-

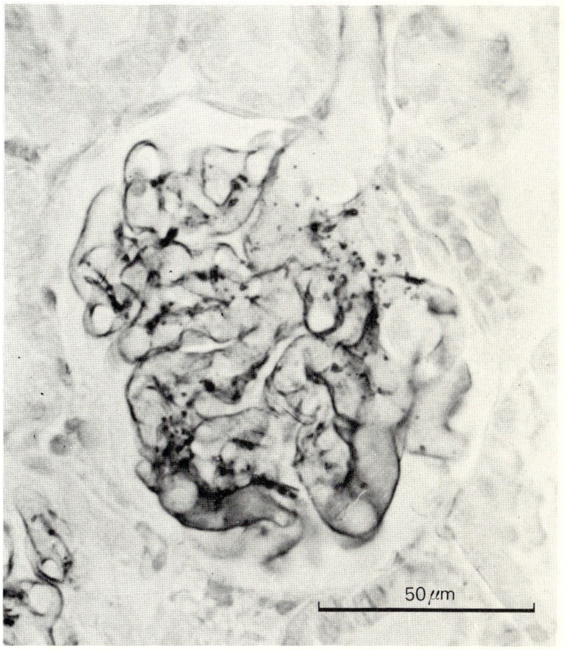

FIG. 6. Photomicrograph of a section of a glomerulus from a rat kidney. The section has not passed through the proximal tubule.

sorbed to a varying extent ("*facultative reabsorption*") so that the final output of urine varies between 0.3 cm^3 and 20 cm^3/min. These figures are approximate and may vary considerably from person to person.

Obligatory reabsorption in the proximal tubule

The study of the functions of the renal tubules has been greatly facilitated by the technique of micropuncture. By means of a micromanipulator, extremely fine hollow glass needles may be used to withdraw fluid from the tubules and blood vessels of the kidney or to inject various foreign substances, the fate of which may then be determined. This technique was first applied to the mammalian kidney by Walker and his colleagues in 1941. Experiments of this kind showed that in the proximal tubule, the reabsorption of water is apparently secondary to the active reabsorption of sodium. Sodium is reabsorbed by the cells and passed into the capillaries, accompanied by appropriate anions (principally chloride) and also by an equivalent amount of water in order to maintain the osmotic equilibrium. Various other substances (such as glucose) are also reabsorbed in the proximal tubule, but the fluid remains isosmotic (*i.e.,* having the same osmolality) with respect to plasma. Therefore, no concentration or dilution of the tubular fluid occurs in this part of the nephron. When such large volumes of filtrate are being dealt with, it is obviously important that the correct amount of salt and water be retrieved

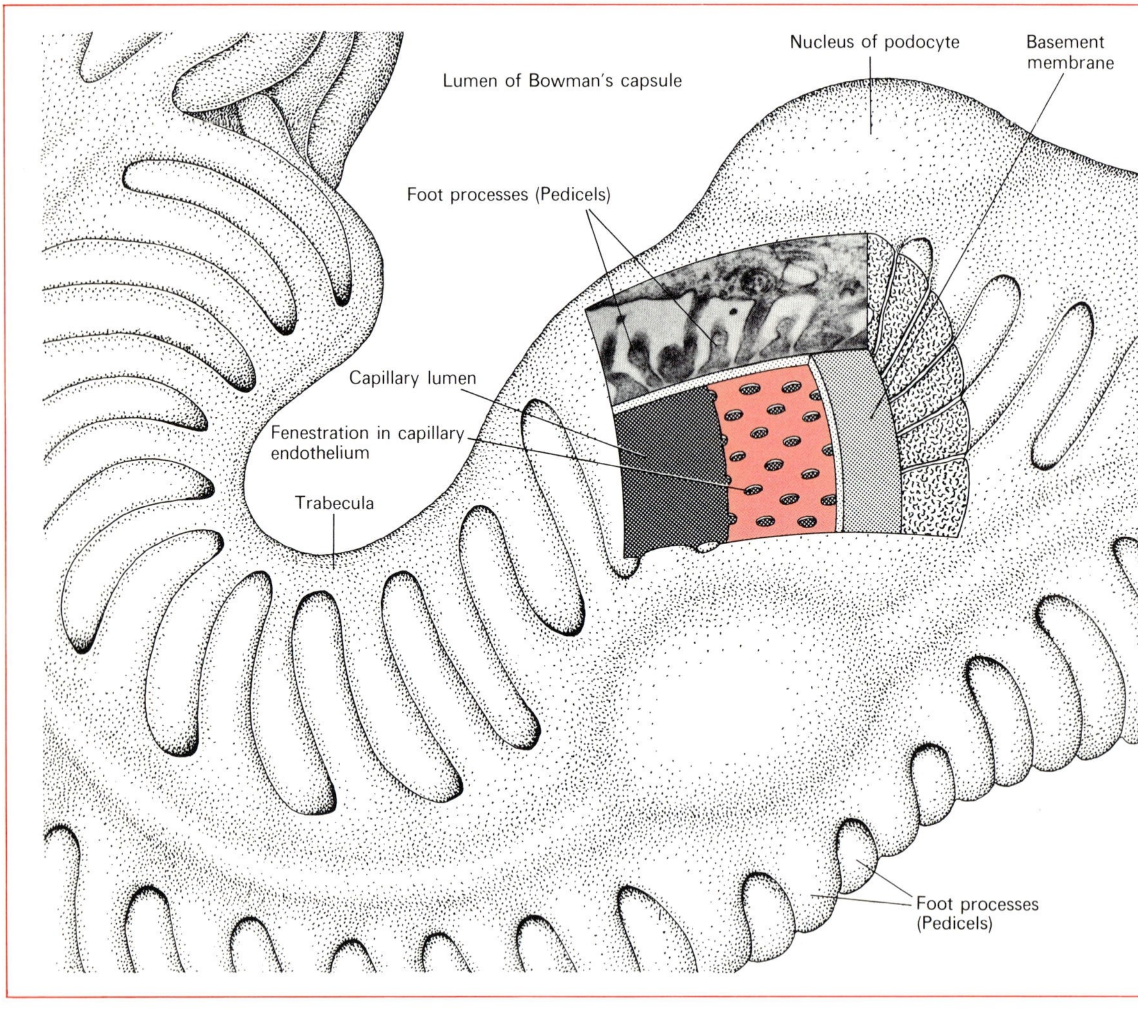

FIG. 7. Diagram to show the interdigitations of the podocytes around a glomerular capillary. The farther side of the "cut-out" is part of the electron micrograph shown in Fig. 8.

from the filtrate. The mechanism that maintains this *"glomerulo-tubular balance"* is the subject of intensive research at present. There is, however, no general consensus of opinion as to its mode of operation so far.

The structure of the proximal tubule reveals something of its functions (Figs. 11, 12, and 13), being typical of cells which are transporting large quantities of solute and water. The area of the inner (luminal) surface of the cells is increased some 36-fold by the presence of a *brush border*. This brush border consists of innumerable microvilli which are bathed on all sides by the tubular fluid. The basal surface area is similarly increased by *basal infoldings* of the cell membrane, each invagination being occupied by a process from an adjacent cell. Associated with the basal cell membrane is a special type of the enzyme, *adenosine triphosphatase* (Na-K-ATPase), which plays an important role in the active transport of sodium out of the cell. The energy required for such active transport is provided by the enzyme activity of the large and numerous mitochondria which are very closely related to the basal infoldings (Fig. 12).

Facultative reabsorption in the distal part of the nephron

It is now known that facultative reabsorption of water is the result of osmotic effects in the most distal part of the nephron and in the collecting ducts of the medulla. It is dependent upon the establishment of an osmotic gradient between the tubular lumen and the surrounding tissues. Earlier theories about the concentration of urine by the continuous reabsorption of water as the glomerular filtrate passes along the tubules became more and more difficult to accept in the light of experimental results. For example, micropuncture studies by Walker and his colleagues indicated that the tubular fluid at the beginning of the distal tubule of the rat is usually hypo-osmotic (*i.e.,* it has an osmolality below that of plasma), even when concentrated urine is being produced.

Another important finding was that of Wirz, Hargitay, and Kuhn in 1951. They investigated the osmolality of the rat renal medulla by utilizing the principle that the osmolality of a solution is closely related to its freezing point. The technique actually used was to find the thawing point of previously frozen slices of kidney. These experi-

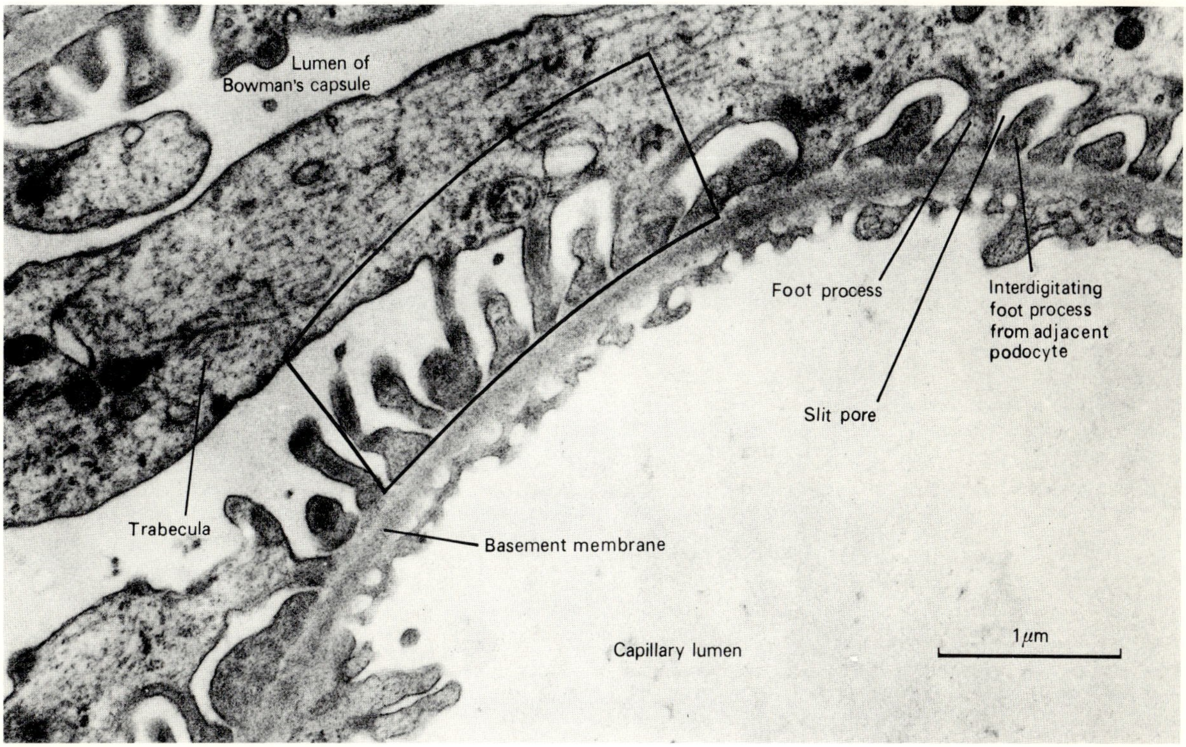

FIG. 8. Electron micrograph of part of a glomerulus from the rat kidney. The quadrilateral area indicates the region of the "cut-out" in Fig. 7.

ments showed that there is an osmotic gradient in the tissues of the medulla, increasing toward the tip of the papilla where the osmolality is up to 8 times that of plasma. Putting these findings together, it seems that the isosmotic (*i.e.*, isosmotic to plasma) fluid which is leaving the proximal tubule becomes more and more concentrated as it descends the loop of Henle. It becomes, however, less and less concentrated again as it ascends the loop until, as it enters the distal tubule, it is hypo-osmotic to plasma. Further clues to the functions of the loop of Henle came from comparative studies. Only birds and mammals are able to produce a concentrated urine, and only they possess a complete Henle's loop. There is also a correlation between the relative thickness of the medulla in different species (Fig. 14) and the ability to produce concentrated urine.

These observations seem to be very puzzling when viewed in isolation, but a theory which fits all the facts had already been advanced before most of the observations had been made. In 1942, Kuhn and Ryffel suggested that a *counter-current multiplication process*, already familiar to physicists, might be applicable to the kidney. This idea is now generally accepted, with some modifications, and current research is largely concerned with determining the exact site and mechanism of the multiplier system.

The principle of counter-current exchange and multiplication

A simple counter-current exchange system is illustrated by the engineer's method of using hot exhaust gas from an engine to heat the incoming air (Fig. 15). As it leaves the engine, the gas is extremely hot, but as it passes along the exhaust tube it rapidly becomes cooler as heat is transferred to the incoming air which is flowing in the opposite direction (hence the use of the term, "counter-current"). The incoming air, therefore, becomes hotter as it approaches the engine. There is thus established a gradient of temperature in which the gas or air in both inlet and exhaust pipes is very hot near the engine, but is almost at atmospheric temperature near the external apertures.

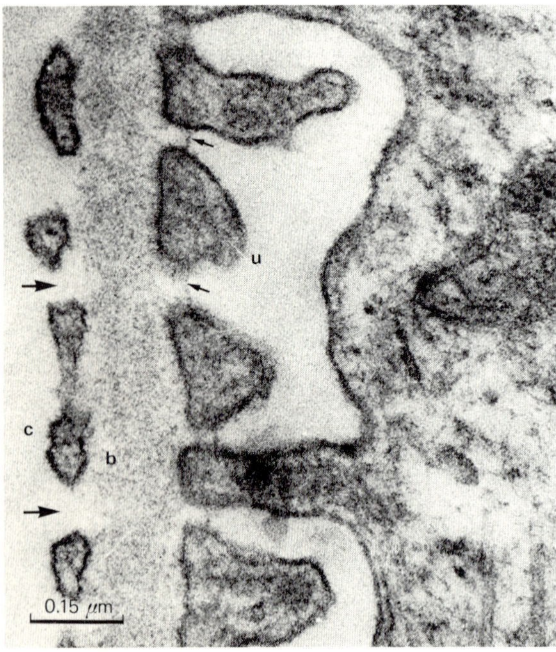

FIG. 9. The membrane between the blood and the cavity of Bowman's capsule. The lumen of the capillary (c) lies to the left; the cavity of Bowman's capsule (u) lies to the right. The endothelium has numerous fenestrations (large arrows). The slit-pores between the foot processes are closed by a thin membrane (small arrows). The principal structure separating blood from glomerular filtrate is the basement membrane (b).

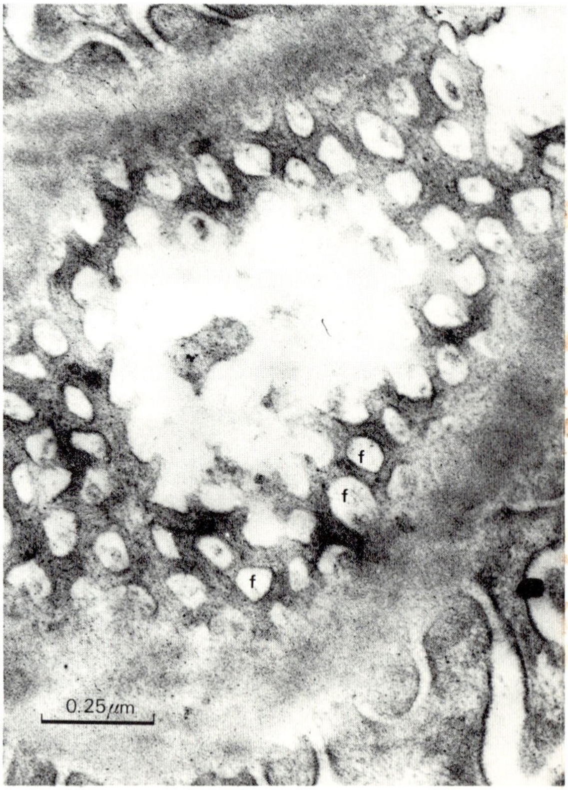

FIG. 10. A tangential section through a glomerular capillary. The endothelial fenestrations (f) are clearly visible.

Heat is thus not dissipated into the atmosphere, but is conserved within the machine. Suppose that, for some extraordinary reason, the exhaust pipe was connected to the inlet pipe (Fig. 15 (b)). Conditions, at least as far as the temperature in the tubes is concerned, would not be greatly al-tered. The cool gas, which previously escaped the air, would now reenter the machine, and be reheated in the process. This would not od idea for engines, but the same principle f a counter-current *exchanger*) is found in iological situations. In aquatic mammals whales, for instance, the warm blood pass- the extremities would dissipate an us amount of body heat into the Arctic re it not for the fact that the main artery of to the limb or flipper is very closely sur- by a large number of veins which return od to the trunk. Heat is transferred from tery to the veins along their length so that is conserved at the body end of the system. these counter-current heat exchange sys-ns, the exchange of heat between the tubes is a passive or "downhill" transfer down a heat gradient; such a system can only conserve the heat which is already present—it cannot build up extra heat. Fig. 15(c) shows a further development of the counter-current principle in which an active or "uphill" transport system takes part. The U-tube is supposed to contain a circulating sodium chloride solution. A mechanism is present which is capable of *actively* transferring sodium (and chloride) ions from the ascending to the descending limb of the U-tube, *without any accompanying water*. As a result of this process, the osmolality of the fluid in the descending limb will increase as it approaches the hairpin bend. After rounding the bend, the highly concentrated fluid will gradually undergo a diminution in osmolality as solute is extruded (without water) until the fluid emerges from the upper end of the tube with an osmolality slightly below that at which it entered the system. When *active* transport occurs, therefore, if the loop is long enough, a very high osmolality can be built up toward the U-bend although at any one level only a small osmotic gradient exists between

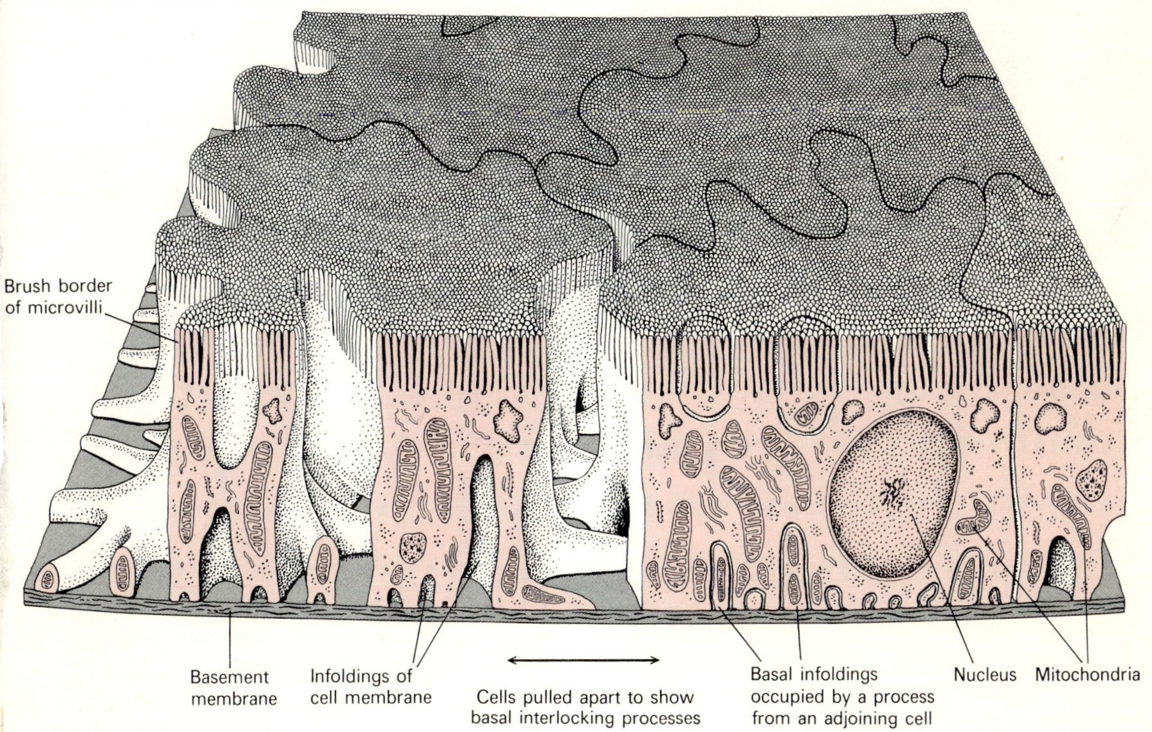

FIG. 11. Diagram to show part of the epithelium of a proximal tubule. Note particularly the brush border and the basal infoldings, each of which is occupied by a process from an adjoining cell. The cells are resting on a basement membrane.

the two tubes. Thus, the "single effect" of a small active transfer of solute at any one level can be multiplied along the length of the tube to produce a large total effect. This is therefore known as a *counter-current multiplier* system. Active transport of sodium ions is sometimes referred to as the *"sodium pump"* and it requires the expenditure of energy (See Chappell, CBR No. 50).

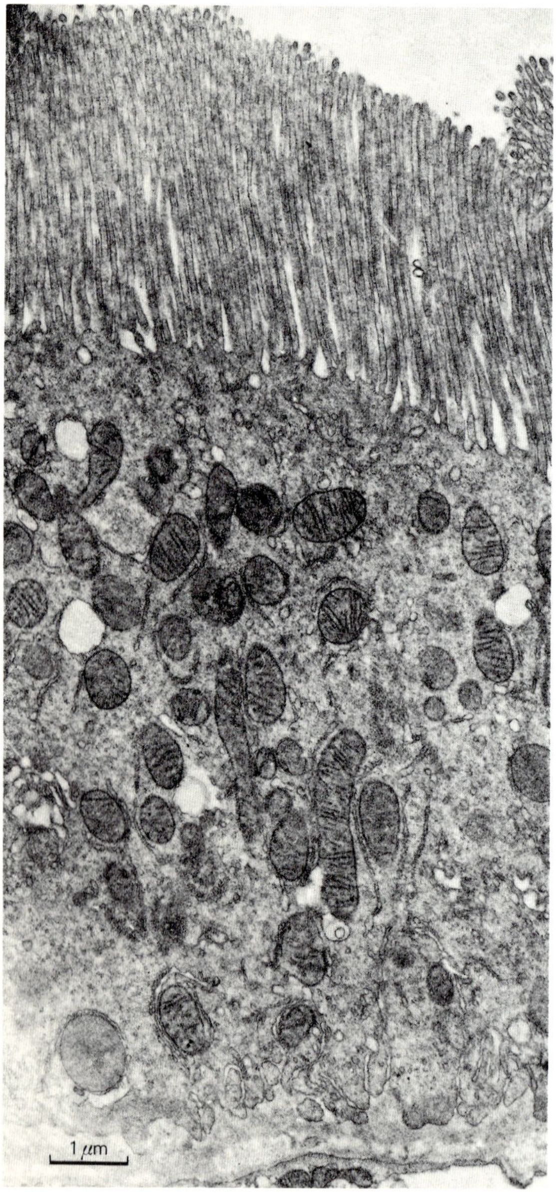

FIG. 12. Electron micrograph of part of a proximal tubule cell from a rat kidney. Note the brush border, the numerous mitochondria, and the basal infoldings. The space at the bottom is a peritubular capillary.

Counter-current multiplication in the loops of Henle

This process, with some modification, forms the basis for the establishment of the osmotic gradient in the medulla of the kidney. The figures for osmolality which are shown in Fig. 15(c) might apply to a loop of Henle. In the loops, sodiu (along with appropriate anions—mostly ride), is actively transported at all levels out ascending limb into the interstitial (intert tissue and then into the descending limb. multiplier system is set up and the lality of the loops of Henle and the int tissue (including the blood vessels) incre ward the tip of the papilla. You will remen the collecting ducts have to travel thro zone of greatly increased osmolality in c pass their contents into the pelvis of the (Fig. 1).

This description is meant only as a guide general principles of counter-current multi tion. The process is almost certainly slightly

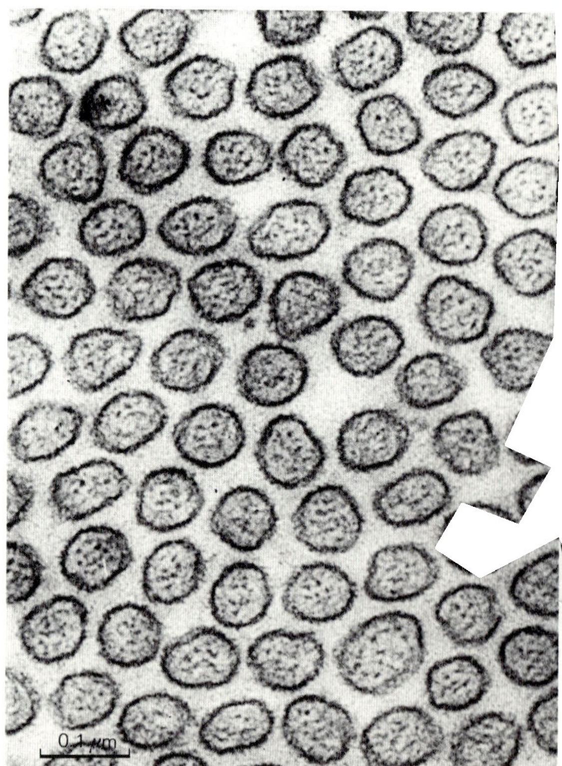

FIG. 13. A transverse section through the brush border of a proximal tubule cell, to show how this greatly increases the surface area of the cell exposed to the tubular fluid.

ferent in the living kidney. For example, recent work has suggested that in the thick part of the ascending limb there is a chloride pump rather than a sodium pump. Also, it is not essential that salt should enter the descending limb. If it is transported from the ascending limb into the interstitial tissue, it would then be able to cause the osmotic extraction of water from the descending limb. This would, thus, concentrate the fluid in the latter without the necessity for the entry of salt. Other alternative systems are mentioned below.

Distal tubules

Further active reabsorption of salt takes place in the distal tubules. The transport process is slightly different from that in the proximal tubule, since here it is controlled by various hormones and is not accompanied by the reabsorption of water. Thus, the contents of the distal tubule become even more hypo-osmotic as they pass along the tubule.

Concentration and dilution of the urine

With this data in mind, it is now possible to understand the mechanism of concentration and dilution of the urine. If the walls of the collecting ducts were freely permeable to water, then water would pass through them into the interstitial tissue. This would occur in the cortical collecting ducts because the contents are hypo-osmotic relative to the surrounding tissues and capillaries, and in the main collecting ducts because the medullary interstitial tissue is hyperosmotic relative to the tubular fluid. Osmotic equilibration will, therefore, demand the transfer of water out of the tubules and the urine will be concentrated. If, on the other hand, the collecting ducts were impermeable to water, the hypo-osmotic fluid entering the collecting duct system would be conducted safely through the medulla with little, if any, loss of water and the urine would be dilute.

The permeability of the collecting ducts is known to be controlled by the antidiuretic hormone (ADH). The excretion of a large amount of dilute urine is known as *diuresis* and the antidiuretic hormone, which is secreted by the pituitary gland in response to the need to conserve water, leads to the production of a concentrated urine by increasing the permeability of the collecting ducts to water. It should, perhaps, be mentioned that, until recently, it was thought that the distal tubule was also responsive to ADH. Current research, however, has indicated that this is probably not so.

Structure of the loops of Henle

Unfortunately, physiological experiments and structural studies do not always lead to the same conclusions, and this is particularly true of the loops of Henle. According to the counter-current multiplication theory, the thin ascending limb of the loop of Henle should be capable of active transport of large quantities of salt. One would therefore expect it to have a structure rather like the proximal tubule. In fact, it is composed of very simple, flattened cells (Fig. 16 (a)) with hardly any mitochondria. On the other hand, the thick ascending limb in the outer medulla has precisely the structure one would expect, with numerous large mitochondria and deep basal infoldings (Fig. 16 (b)). Various explanations of the counter-current mechanism have now been put forward in which all the active transport of salt occurs in this region of the loop.

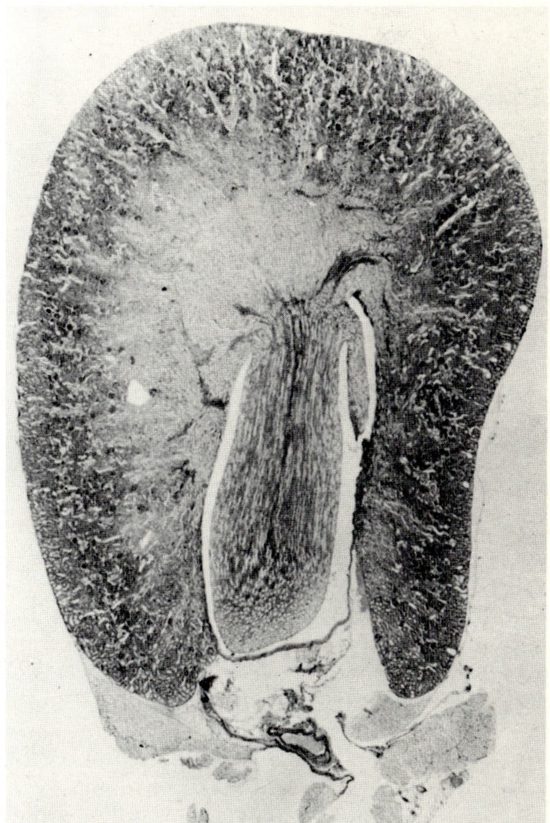

FIG. 14. Transverse section through the kidney of a desert rodent *(Gerbillus)*. Note the extremely long papilla.

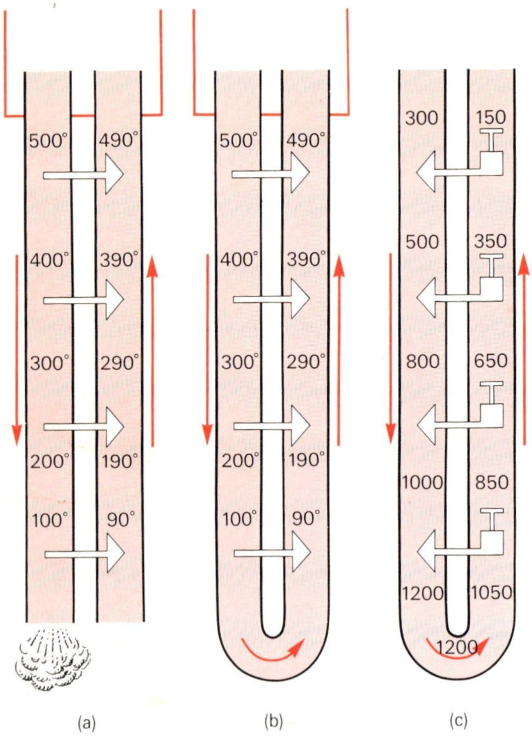

FIG. 15. Diagrams to represent (a) heating of incoming air by exhaust gas in an engine; in practice a large number of tubes are used to increase the surface area available for heat exchange; (b) a counter-current heat exchange system; and (c) a counter-current *multiplier* system involving the *active* transport of sodium from the ascending limb to the descending limb, by means of a "sodium pump." This has the effect of building up a high osmolality (expressed in mosmol/kg) toward the U-bend, although at any one level there is only a small difference in osmolality between the two limbs.

In addition, it is known that one of the waste products of the body—urea—plays an important part in producing the osmotic gradient in the medulla. This, too, is probably involved in a counter-current system. For example, Kokko and Rector have suggested that active transport of salt out of the thick ascending limb (and later, out of the distal tubule) renders the tubular fluid hypotonic relative to the surrounding interstitial fluid. Water is, therefore, extracted from the cortical collecting duct system, leading to a high intratubular concentration of urea. This urea passes from the inner medullary collecting ducts into the medullary interstitium. This causes the removal of water from the descending limbs of the loops of Henle which, in turn, increases their sodium concentration. After rounding the bend, sodium in the ascending limbs therefore passes (passively) out into the interstitium, rendering the intratubular fluid hypotonic. Both sodium ions and urea, therefore, contribute to the medullary osmotic gradient. This and other recent theories call for particular permeability properties of the tubules. At present these theories are still being investigated. Thus, at this time, there is no generally agreed upon theory of the precise mechanism of the counter-current multiplier system.

The medullary blood vessels

It is probable that counter-current multiplication in the loops of Henle is not the only factor concerned in building up and maintaining the osmotic gradient of the medulla. The anatomical peculiarities of the blood supply to the medulla suggest that the blood vessels may play an important part. The efferent arterioles of the glomeruli nearest to the medulla—the *juxtamedullary glomeruli*—follow a course different from that of the efferent arterioles of the more superficial glomeruli. After leaving the glomerulus, the efferent arteriole passes into the medulla and breaks up into a leash of vessels known as *descending vasa recta* (Fig. 17). These supply capillary networks in the medulla and from the capillaries, *ascending vasa recta* pass back toward the cortex where they join some of the larger veins (Fig. 2). In the outer medulla, the descending and ascending vasa recta are gathered together to form *vascular bundles* in which the two types of vessel are intermingled and come into close apposition (Fig. 18). Electron microscopy shows that in the bundles the ascending and descending vessels are separated by little more than a very thin layer of interstitial tissue and at most, the thickness of only one cell lies between them (Fig. 19). Structurally, this arrangement is obviously well suited to a counter-current exchange mechanism. For example, the transfer of water from descending to ascending vasa recta in the outer medulla would exclude a certain amount of water from the inner medulla. This would help to maintain the osmotic gradient. Similarly, transfer of solute from ascending to descending vasa recta would recirculate the solute to the inner medulla and, again, contribute to the osmotic gradient. There is a certain amount of evidence that both these processes occur but, so far, no absolute proof is available, part of the difficulty lying in the inaccessibility of this region of the kidney.